LITTLE BOOK OF
REFLEXOLOGY

LITTLE BOOK OF
REFLEXOLOGY

First published in the UK in 2013

© Demand Media Limited 2013

www.demand-media.co.uk

Printed and bound in Europe.

ISBN 978-1-782811-86-2

The views in this book are those of the author but they are general views only and readers are urged to consult the relevant and qualified specialist for individual advice in particular situations.

Demand Media Limited hereby exclude all liability to the extent permitted by law of any errors or omissions in this book and for any loss, damage or expense (whether direct or indirect) suffered by a third party relying on any information contained in this book.

All our best endeavours have been made to secure copyright clearance for every photograph used but in the event of any copyright owner being overlooked please address correspondence to Demand Media Limited, Waterside Chambers, Bridge Barn Lane, Woking, Surrey, GU21 6NL

In no way will Demand Media Limited or any persons associated with Demand Media be held responsible for any injuries or problems that may occur during the use of this book or the advise contained within. We recommend that you consult a doctor before embarking any exercise programme. This product is for informational purposes only and is not meant as medical advice. Performing exercise of all types can pose a risk, know your physical limits, we suggest you perform adequate warm up and cool downs before and after any exercise. If you experience any pain, discomfort, dizziness or become short of breath stop exercising immediately and consult your doctor.

Contents

Introduction

Some sources suggest that foot reflexology originated in Peru in about the 12th century B.C. The technique was also practiced in China and in India more than 5,000 years ago, as well as in Ancient Egypt. It wasn't until the 1930s thanks to the work of American physiotherapist Eunice Ingham, however, that reflexology obtained its present day status, with a foot chart reflecting the whole body.

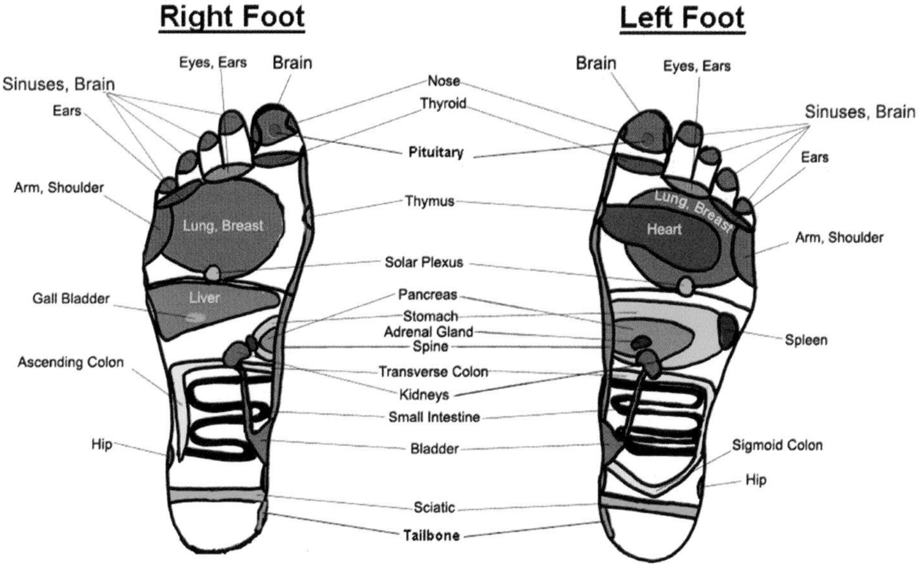
Right Foot
Left Foot
Eyes, Ears
Brain
Sinuses, Brain
Ears
Arm, Shoulder
Lung, Breast
Gall Bladder
Liver
Ascending Colon
Hip
Nose
Thyroid
Pituitary
Thymus
Solar Plexus
Pancreas
Stomach
Adrenal Gland
Spine
Transverse Colon
Kidneys
Small Intestine
Bladder
Sciatic
Tailbone
Brain
Eyes, Ears
Sinuses, Brain
Ears
Lung, Breast
Heart
Arm, Shoulder
Spleen
Sigmoid Colon
Hip

The aim of the Little Book of Reflexology is to teach you how to use the technique to treat the ailments and pains of those around you. It will explain the different reference points on the foot so that you can locate the various zones to be treated.

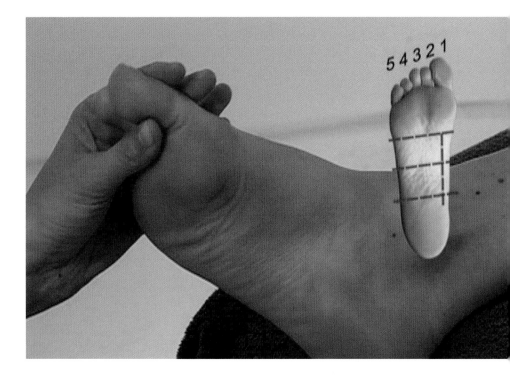

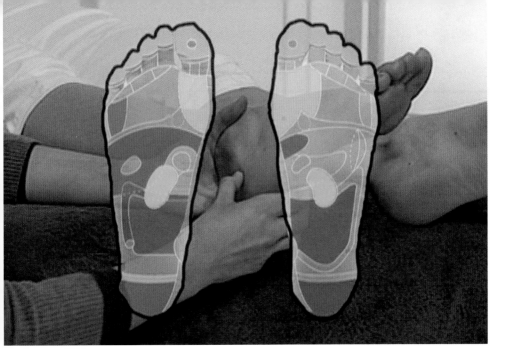

Foot reflexology is an ancient science that considers that the feet mirror the body. Specific areas on the feet, known as reflex zones, correspond to individual organs, glands or parts of the body. The technique works on the oriental principle of dividing the body into longitudinal zones called meridians. Meridians are channels that carry energy to all parts of the human body and they all terminate in the feet. According to this principle, each part of the body is represented by a specific reflex zone found in the foot.

There are different lines that divide up the foot. First there is the diaphragm line, which is situated at the junction of the metatarsals and the phalanges.

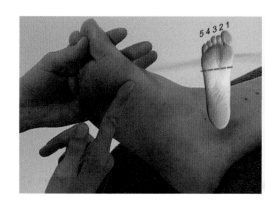

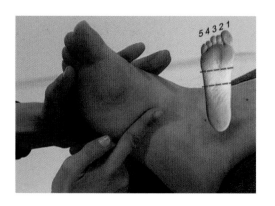

Then there's the waistline, which is a horizontal line beginning at the base of the fifth metatarsal.

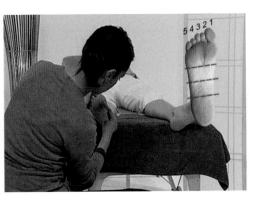

The heel line is found at the bottom of the foot arch where the skin on the heel is at its thickest.

Finally there's the ligaments line found in zone 1 underneath the big toe; it can easily be identified by turning the big toe up.

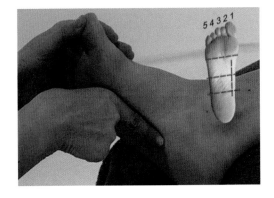

Chapter 1

Basic Foot Reflexology Technique

The basic technique used in foot reflexology is a creeping movement in which the inside of the thumb is placed flat and the fleshy part of the thumb moves forwards like a caterpillar movement. The thumb is kept at an angle of 45 degrees and should not go backwards, move in circles, or slide along. It has to constantly work forward.

Step 1

Step 2

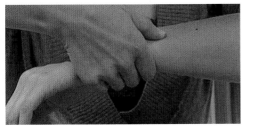

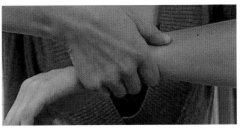

Step 3

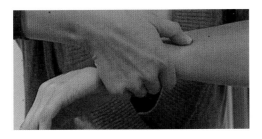

The technique of applying pressure can also be used in foot reflexology. The thumb is kept quite still and used to exert pressure on a precise point on the foot. The amount of pressure should be carefully controlled. If it is too weak it will have no effect, but if the pressure is too strong and causes pain to the patient, it doesn't work either. The pressure should be consistent and adapted to each person.

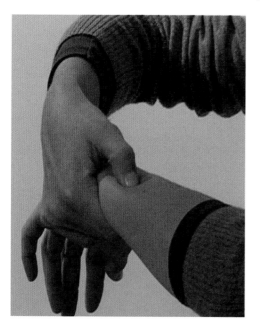

The thumb of the hand doing the work should remain in contact with the skin at all times, while the other hand should be used to support the foot.

Before beginning a session, make sure that your hands are really warm; cold hands can upset the patient.

Begin with some relaxation movements: the first moves forward and back. The hands are placed on either side of the metatarsals and they travel rapidly forwards and back. This doesn't just make the foot and ankle move, but also affects the leg right up to the hip. This movement can be made as the ankle is relaxed.

Step 1

Step 2

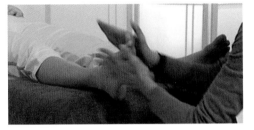

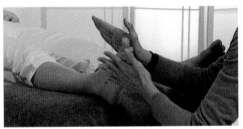

Step 3

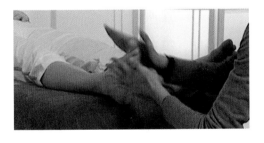

The palms of both hands are then placed on the ankle bones and are pressed down quite hard so as not to cause any chaffing. The hands then move front to back, but should never rotate.

Step 1

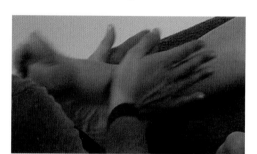

Step 2

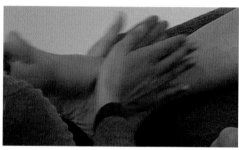

Step 3

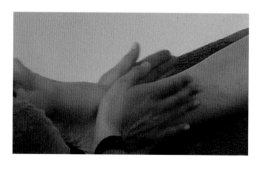

Finally, one other relaxation movement at the start of a session is the rotation of the ankle. Holding the heel firmly with one hand, place the other hand level with the junction between the phalanges and the metatarsals. Rotate the foot in one direction and then in the other.

Step 1

Step 2

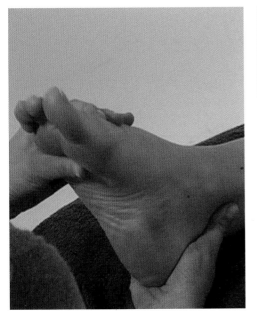

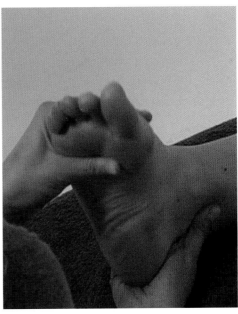

Any combination of relaxation movements at the start of a session should not last longer than five minutes. Their aim is to get the patient to relax and let go, so that he or she is ready for the reflexology session. Relaxation movements are carried out on one foot and then on the other. They also give the practitioner the opportunity to see if there are any areas on the foot that are thicker, reddened or more delicate or swollen. These are indications of where the most sensitive areas on the feet are, and these zones will correspond to parts of the body that have been weakened or are congested.

Chapter 2

The Respiratory System

First looking at the respiratory system, the first zone to work on will be the nose. This zone is found on the big toe and more specifically, on the central third of the big toe.

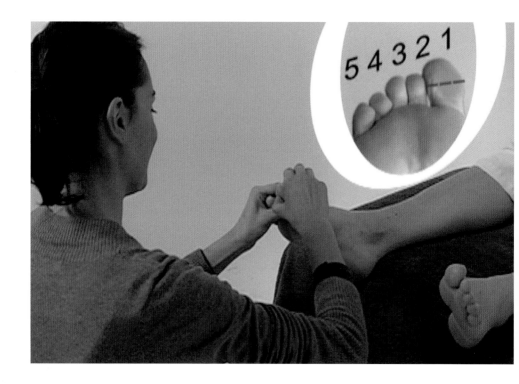

This is worked by using creeping thumb movements, moving inwards from the outer edge and then moving out to the edge from the inside. If particular attention is required in this area then the treatment can last for up to five or six minutes.

Step 1

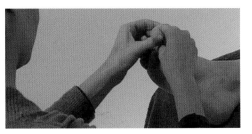

Step 2

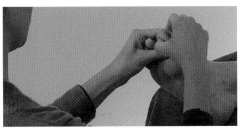

Step 3

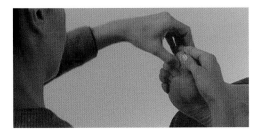

Once work on a particular zone is finished, a relaxation movement is carried out. With regard to the nose, this consists of smoothing the big toe using both thumbs. Two or three movements are enough.

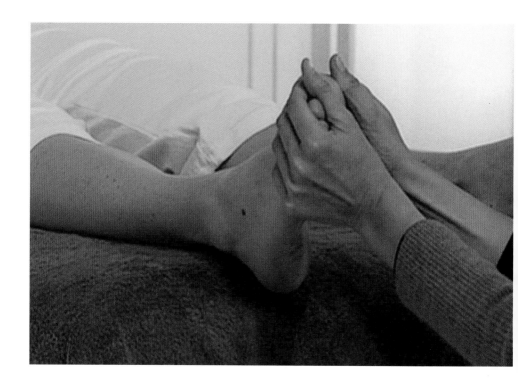

The sinuses are the next area for treatment and the zones for these correspond with the fleshy part of each toe. These are worked on from top to bottom and from the middle to the outer edge. Move out and then back.

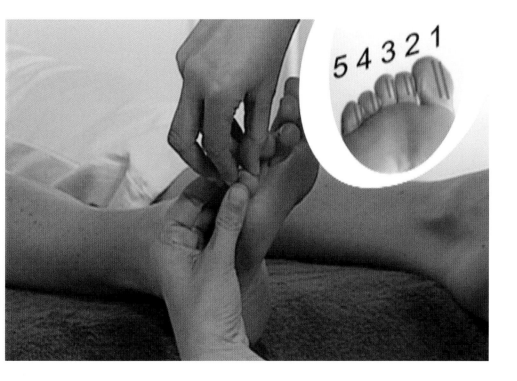

The reflex zone for the throat is situated at the base of the big toe and is treated using creeping movements. Move out and back from the inner edge to the outer edge or vice versa.

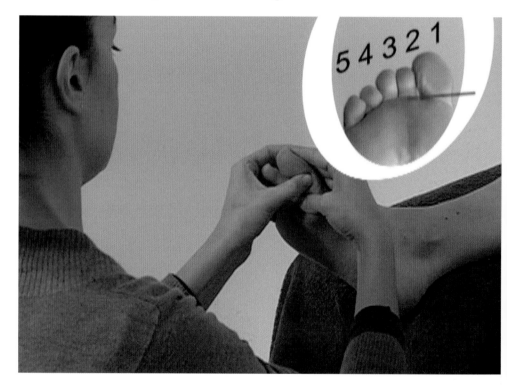

Vertical movements can also be used going either from bottom to top, or from top to bottom.

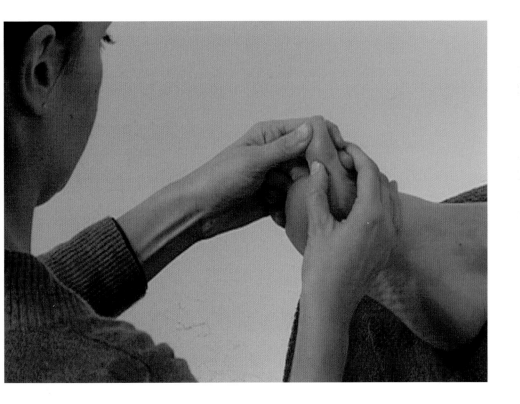

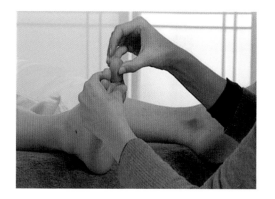

The reflex zone for the throat can be relaxed by rotating the big toe; two or three times is enough.

The bronchi zone can be found both on the sole and the top of the foot.

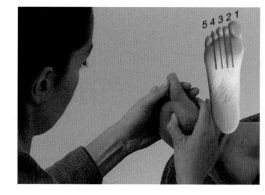

Start with the zone on the sole running over each furrow between the diaphragm line and the base of the toes.

Step 1

Step 2

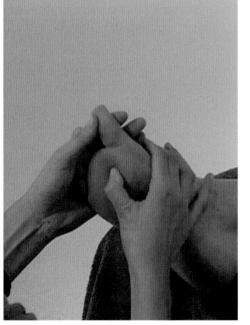
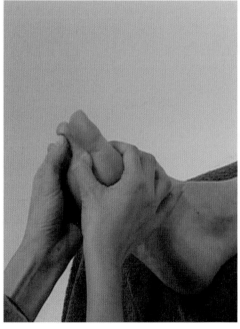

The basic thumb technique is always used on the sole of the foot and it is necessary to run over each reflex zone several times. To make it easier to identify the furrows on the sole of the foot, it is sometimes a good idea to pull the toes apart to make the furrow more prominent.

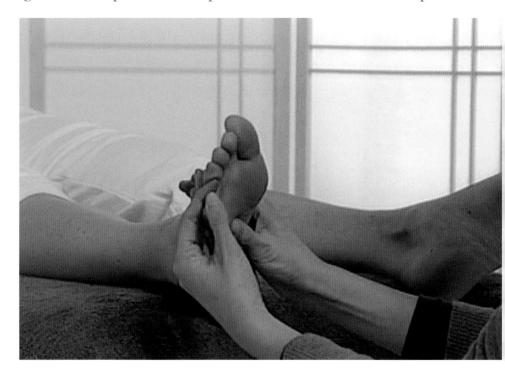

Relaxation of the bronchi is done by massaging the deep intermetatarsal tissue. Both hands are placed flat, facing one another, level with the metatarsals. The deep tissue muscle is moved by the pressure applied using both hands. Very slow circular movements are then made by each hand in turn. These can move in one direction at first, and then the other. As with any other reflex zone, relaxation movements should not last more than one minute.

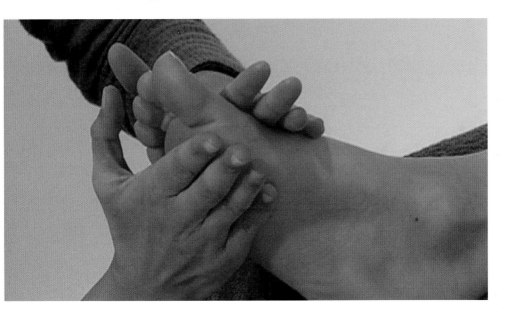

Having worked on the sole of the foot, the bronchi reflex zone on the top of the foot can be worked on.

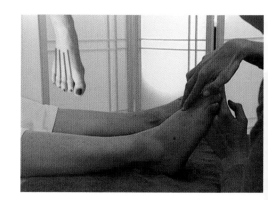

The same creeping movement is used but working with the index finger this time. The foot is held in the other hand so that the metatarsals are stretched as much as possible.

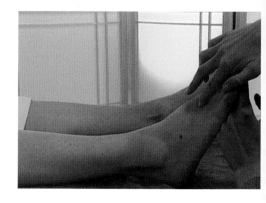

Work on the bronchi reflex zone is used in cases of bronchitis, nicotine intoxication, or withdrawal symptoms, as well as other respiratory problems.

The reflex zone for the lungs is also found on both the sole and the top of the foot.

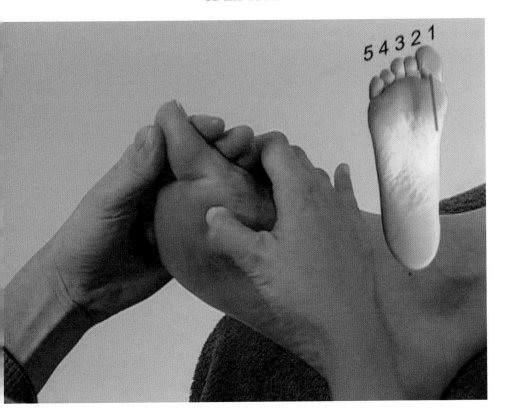

Work starts with the sole again, the reflex zone being between the base of the toes and the diaphragm line across the whole foot. The thumb is used and crosses from bottom to top, moving from the diaphragm line towards the base of the toes; you can go from the outer to the inner edge or the other way, it doesn't matter. One movement out and back will usually be enough, unless there is a specific problem here, and then several movements are required.

Step 1

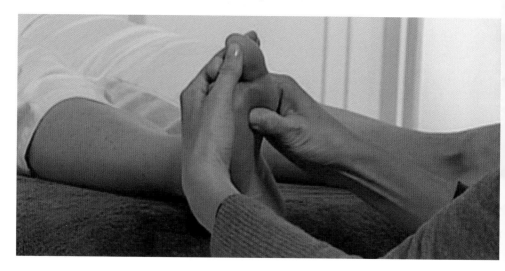

Step 2

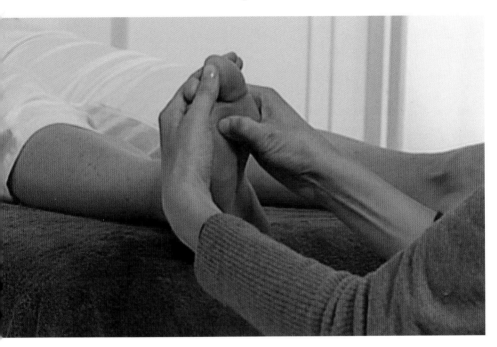

The reflex zone for the lungs should be treated for coughs, asthma, nicotine intoxication or withdrawal symptoms. It can also be used for cases of insomnia, stress and skin problems such as eczema.

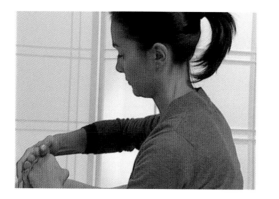

Petrissage of the metatarsals is used to relax the reflex zone of the lungs. Using the top of the hand, the whole metatarsal area on the patient's foot is compressed.

The reflex zone for the lungs is also found on the top of the foot between the base of the toes and the diaphragm line.

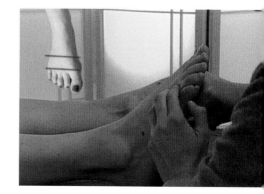

Creeping movements using four fingers are used to treat it this time, moving horizontally from the inside edge to the outer edge, and from the outer edge to the inside edge, constituting one outward and back movement.

Step 1

Step 2

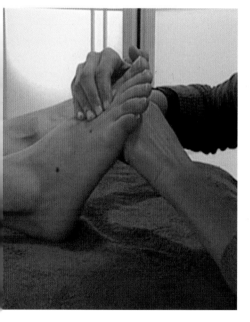

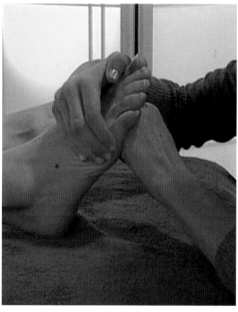

Relaxation of the reflex zone for the lungs on the top of the foot is the same one used for the work on the sole.

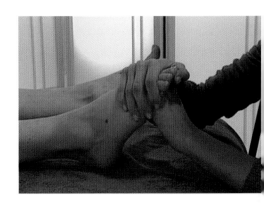

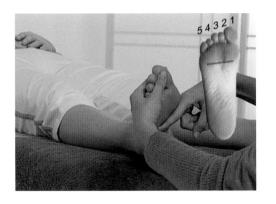

The reflex zone relating to the diaphragm itself is found along the diaphragm line that was pointed out at the beginning of this chapter.

Creeping thumb movements from one side to the other, going forwards and then back, are used to treat the diaphragm. Only one forward and back movement is necessary, unless there is a particular need to work on this reflex zone. This is the treatment for stopping hiccups, but it can also be used to relax a person who is stressed.

Step 1

Step 2

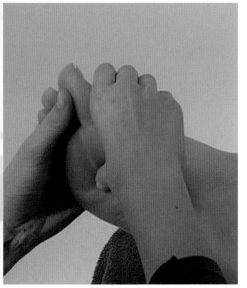
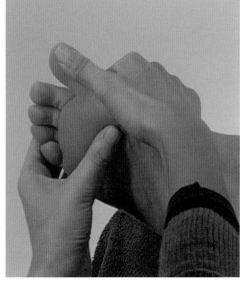

To relax the zone, both thumbs are placed in the middle of the diaphragm line and the foot is opened up. This is done three or four times.

Step 1

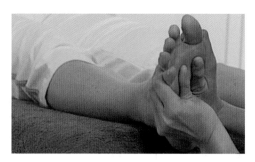

Step 2

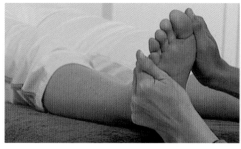

Step 3

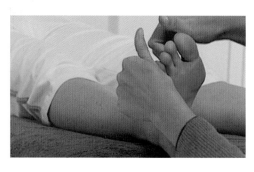

A similar movement is made using the fingers on the top of the foot, and again this is done three or four times.

Step 1

Step 2

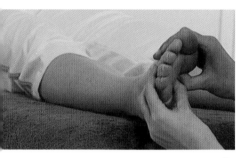

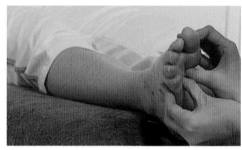

Step 3

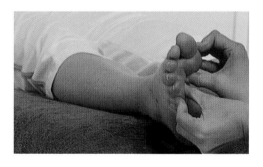

Chapter 3

The Endocrinal System

Work on the endocrinal system begins with work on the reflex zone relating to the pituitary gland, which is more or less in the middle of the big toe at its widest point.

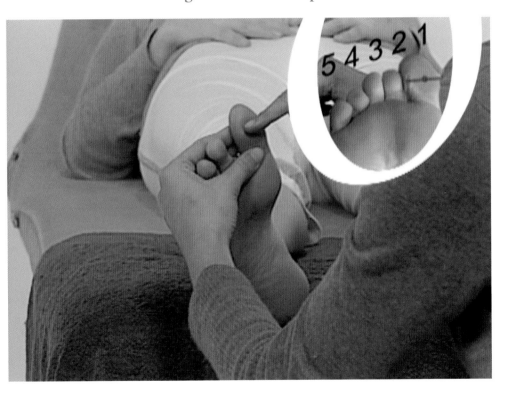

The pituitary gland reflex zone is worked in a fan-shaped motion, starting at the reflex zone you move towards the sides and then up the big toe. The pituitary gland is extremely important, in that it orchestrates the entire endocrinal system, controlling the function of all the other endocrinal glands. It secretes hormones that influence growth, sexuality and pregnancy, as well as water retention and the body's energy levels. This area can be worked if the patient suffers from eating disorders such as anorexia.

Step 1

Step 2

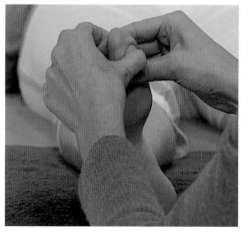
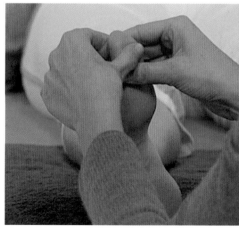

Both thumbs are used to smooth and relax this zone.

Step 1

Step 2

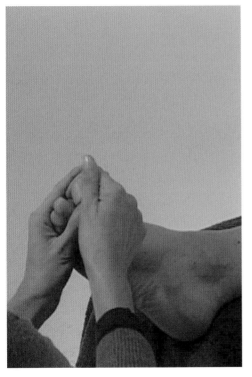
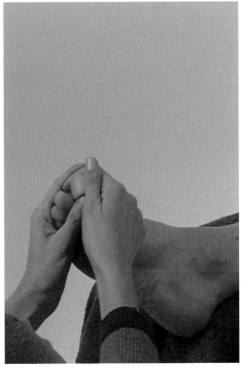

The reflex zone relating to the thyroid is found at the base of the big toe.

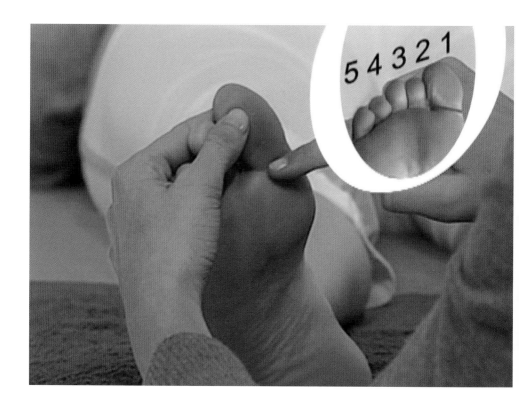

This is in fact the same reflex zone as the throat, and the same method is used as for the pituitary gland in that the movements are made forwards and then back from one edge to the other. The difference is that in this case the movements forward and back are repeated for a second time.

Step 1

Step 2

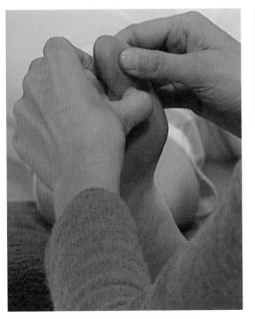

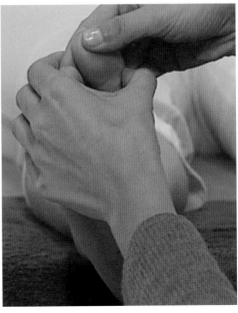

This reflex zone is also worked from the top of the foot. The index finger is used in a forward and back movement.

Step 1

Step 2

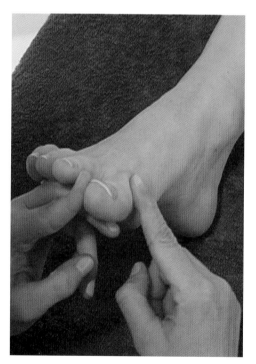
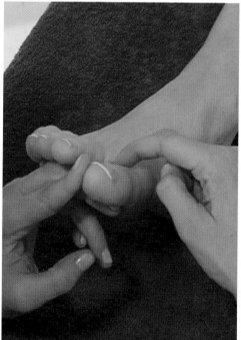

The reflex zone for the adrenal glands is situated on the inner side of the ligament line, approximately at the junction between the lower and middle third of the space between the waist and the diaphragm lines. Thumb pressure is used on this zone. If you press too hard it is not effective; this zone is very sensitive.

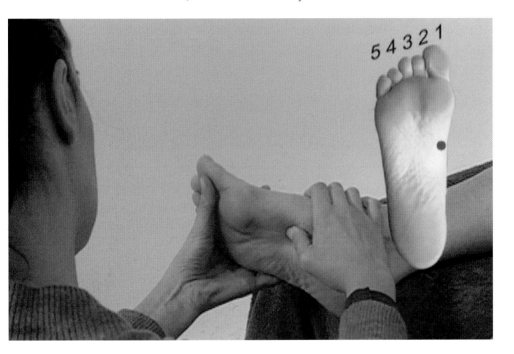

If you have difficulty locating this zone, you can simply run along the inside edge of the ligament line between the waist and the diaphragm lines. Don't be afraid to ask the patient to tell you when you've reached the most sensitive point. The adrenal glands are also called the stress glands, since one of their functions is the secretion of adrenaline. It therefore follows that this is the reflex zone to treat people who are nervous, stressed or suffering from anxiety.

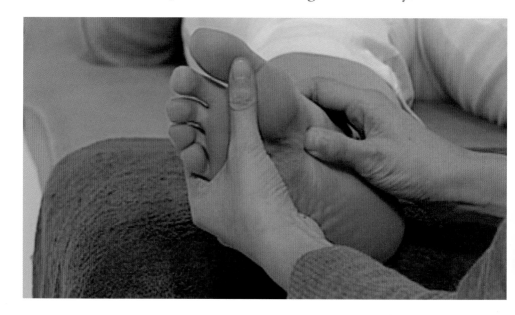

To relax this zone, massage the foot arch by holding the heel with your fingers and supporting the foot with your other hand.

Step 1   Step 2

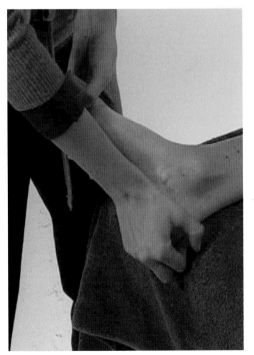

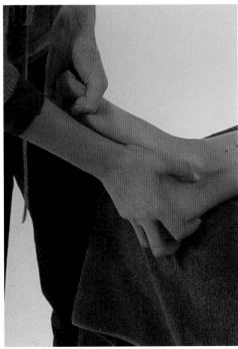

A pancreas reflex zone is present in both feet. The smaller of the two zones is found in zone one on the right foot, zone one being the zone of the big toe. It is situated on a level with the waist line and a little below it. This zone corresponds to the top part of the pancreas.

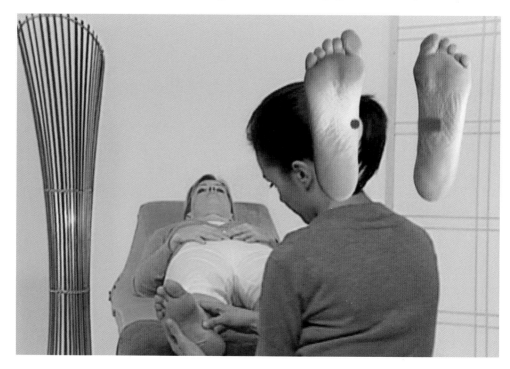

Creeping movements are used, moving from bottom to top and from one side to the other. This small section of the pancreas is of particular interest because it has an endocrinal role. The pancreas plays a role in sugar metabolism through the secretion of insulin and this increases the amount of glucose absorbed by the cells. Amateurs should obviously not attempt to treat the pancreas reflex zone on a person suffering from diabetes.

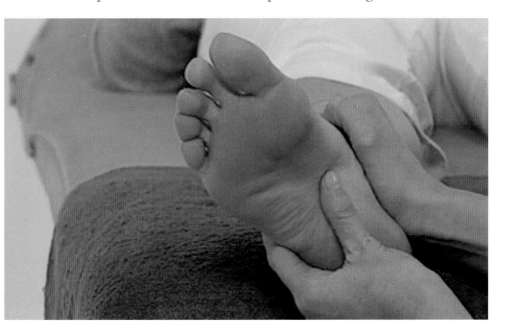

Relaxation of the zone can be achieved by massaging the foot arch, holding the heel with the fingers and supporting the foot with the other hand.

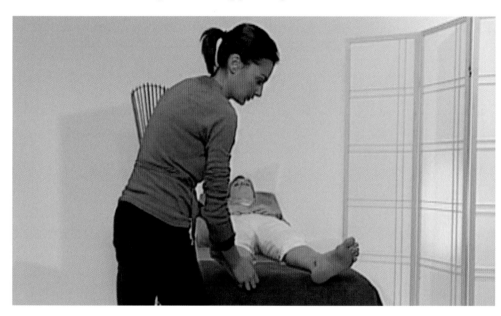

Having completed all of the above techniques, the other foot then has to be treated in the same way as the first one going over all the reflex zones relating to the glands that have been treated so far. The sensations felt by one foot will be very different from those felt by the other.

Note: the pancreas reflex zone is not situated in the same place on both feet. On the left foot it is found half way between the waist line and the diaphragm line.

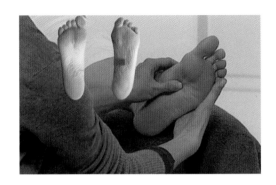

Work is carried out using creeping thumb movements from bottom to top, moving from the waist line to the diaphragm line.

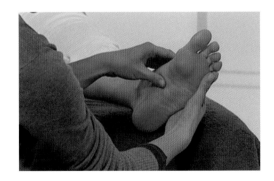

The group of reflex zones relating to the endocrinal system should be treated in cases of hormonal irregularities: hot flushes and sterility. In such cases the reflex zone relating to the uterus and the ovaries should also be treated.

Chapter 4

The Genital System

The reflex zone for the uterus is found on the inside of the ankle. The point is quite precise being at the centre of the line linking the angle of the heel and the top of the anklebone on the inside.

Step 1

Step 2

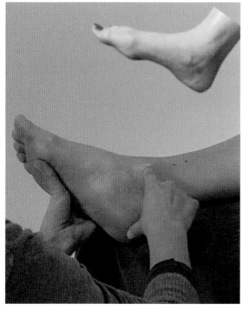

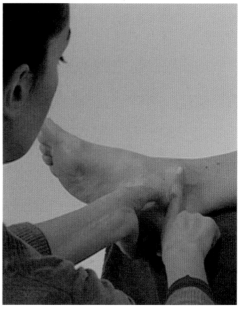

Small creeping movements with the thumb in a star shape are used to treat this sensitive zone; it is ineffective therefore if you press too hard.

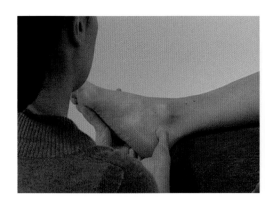

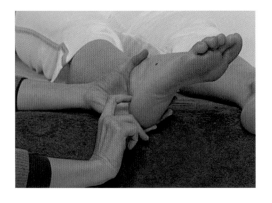

The reflex zone for the ovaries or testicles is situated on the outer surface of the ankle. The exact point is found at the middle of the line linking the angle of the heel on the top of the anklebone.

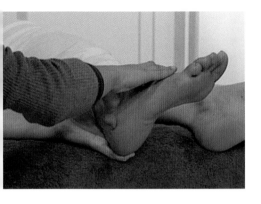

This zone is also treated with the thumb making small star-shaped movements. This is a zone that should not be treated if the patient is pregnant. These zones should be worked on for a little bit longer in cases of sterility. The work stimulates the function of the ovaries.

Relaxation is achieved by rotating the ankle.

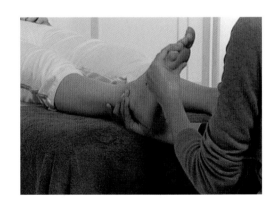

The reflex zone relating to the fallopian tubes and the drainage channels is a line linking the top of the two anklebones above the ankle.

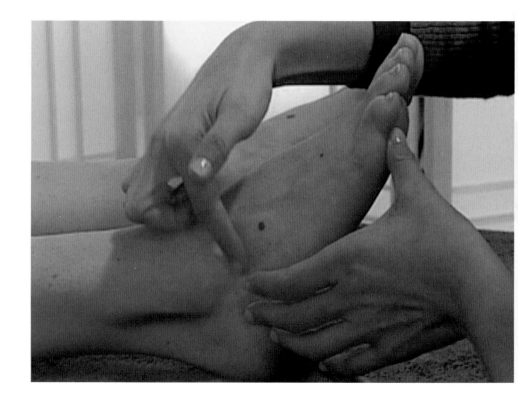

This zone is treated using the index fingers, one index finger moving towards the other just above the ankle. The basic technique is still one of creeping finger movements. During the movement, the thumbs keep the foot in a bent position. The genital system is treated in cases of sterility, ovarian cists, or in the case of men, proctalgia or impotence.

Carry out several forward and back movements in this zone.

Step 1

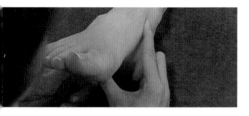

Step 2

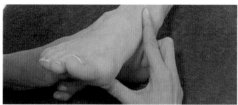

Step 3

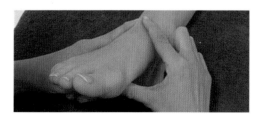

A suitable relaxation movement for this reflex zone is by rotation of the ankle.

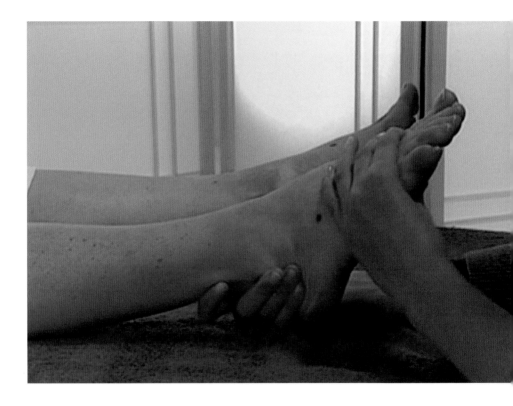

Chapter 5

The Lymphatic System

The first reflex zone relating to the lymphatic system is the thoracic reflex zone. It is treated in the same way as the reflex zone relating to the bronchi – on the top of the foot and the furrows. But this time all the fingers work together using the same creeping movements.

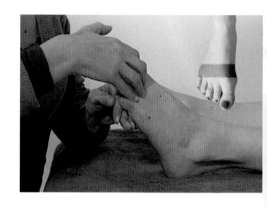

The foot is supported by the other hand that hold it where the toes join the metatarsals, so that the foot is stretched out and the fingers can traverse each furrow.

Step 1

Step 2

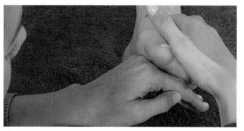

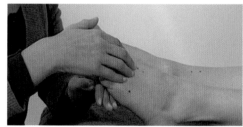

This zone corresponds to the region of the breasts and the lungs – a zone that is rich in lymphatic nodes. The furrows all need to be worked several times and you can go over them ten times.

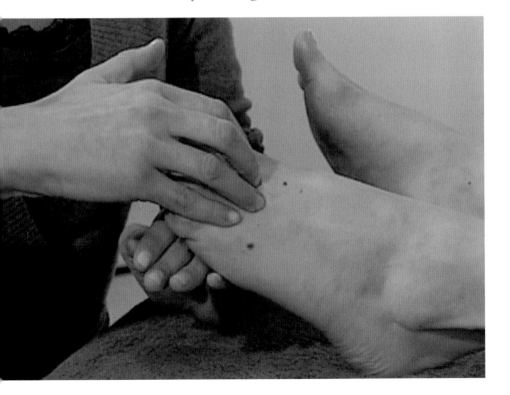

The relaxation movement is the same as the one used to relax the lungs and the bronchi.

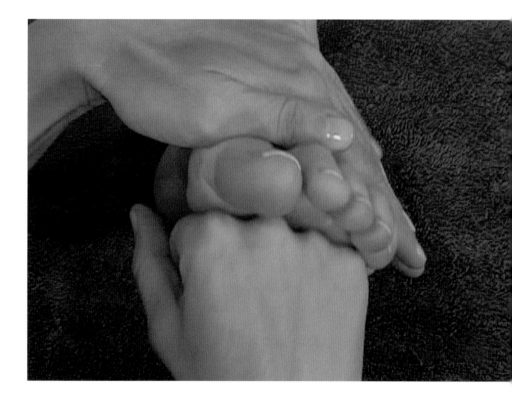

The reflex zone for lymph nodes in the groin is also the reflex zone for the fallopian tubes and the drainage channels. It is a line linking the two anklebones on top of the ankle.

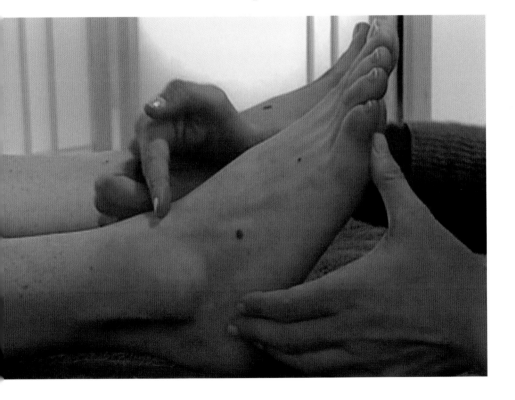

Both index fingers are used at the same time on this area with the thumbs keeping the foot in its bent position. The lymphatic system is an important part of the immune system, since it plays a role in draining away numerous toxins. It is also beneficial to work on this reflex zone for cases of water retention.

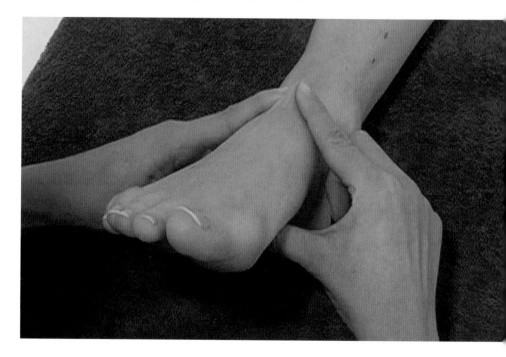

The method used to relax the lymphatic node reflex zone is the same method as that of the fallopian tubes and the drainage channels by rotating the ankle.

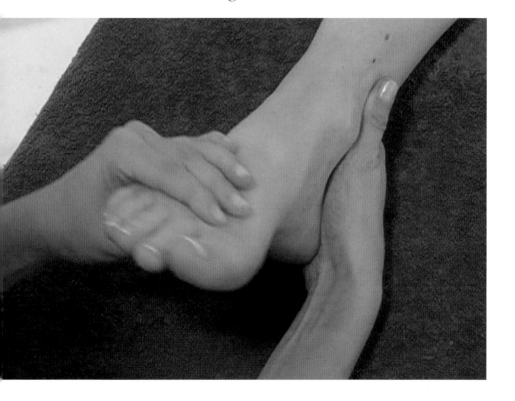

Chapter 6

The Digestive System

The oesophagus reflex zone is worked from top to bottom. The movement begins at the base of the toes and the thumb then moves in creeping movements towards the diaphragm line. One or two forward and backward movements are carried out.

Step 1

Step 2

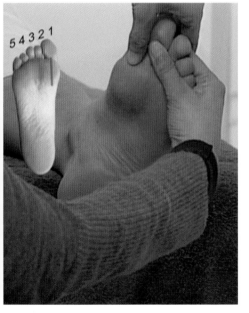 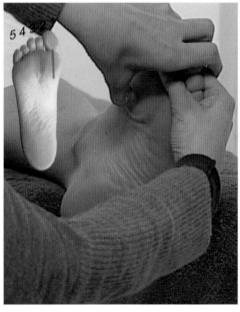

This can be followed by exerting pressure on the point where the oesophagus reflex zone crosses the diaphragm line. This point corresponds to the hernia point.

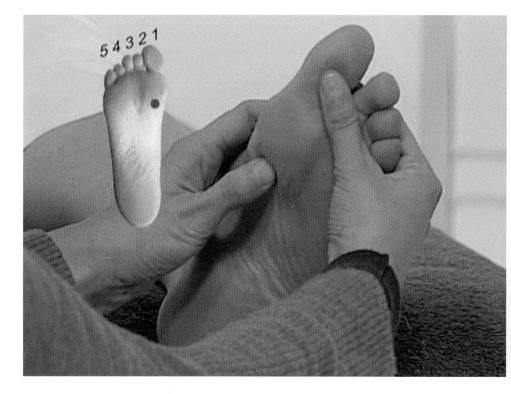

The stomach reflex zone is on the left foot between the diaphragm line and zones one to four of the waist line. Creeping thumb movements crossing diagonally between the waist line towards the diaphragm line are used to treat this zone. Treatment of the stomach and oesophagus reflex zones is useful in cases of flatulence. Note that the stomach's reflex zone is only found on the left foot because the stomach is located on the left side of the body.

Step 1

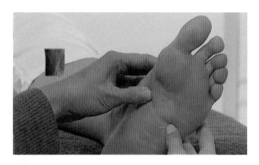

Step 2

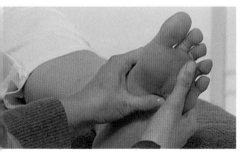

Step 3

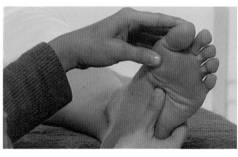

Relaxation of this zone is achieved by massaging the foot arch.

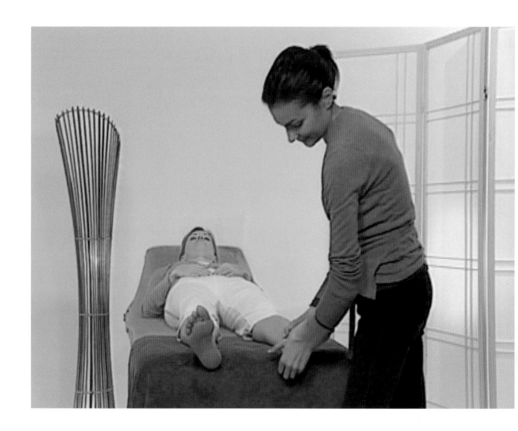

The liver's reflex zone is found on the right foot across the whole zone between the diaphragm line and the waist line.
Creeping thumb movements from the waist line towards the diaphragm line are used to treat this area, moving from one side of the foot to the other.

Step 1

Step 2

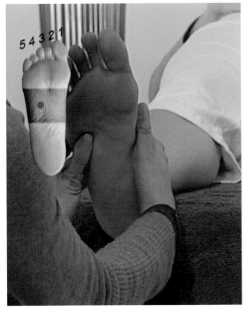

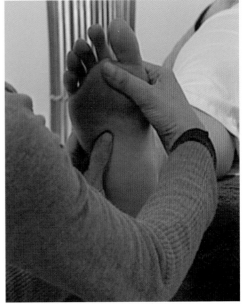

Half way between these two lines and between zones three and four is the reflex zone of the bile duct. Thumb pressure is used on this point. This zone can be quite tender in people suffering from problems related to the digestion.

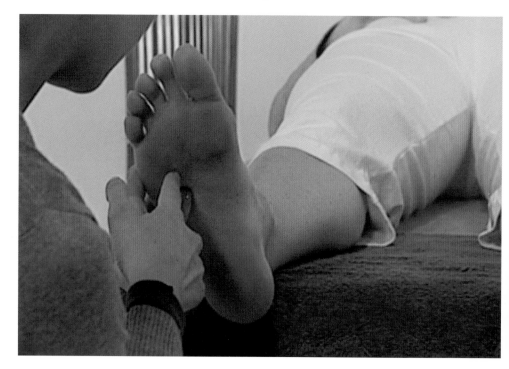

When the bile duct reflex zone has been well worked, work begins again on the liver's reflex zone. On returning to work in this zone, however, a pause is made this time on that of the bile duct before continuing.

Step 1

Step 2

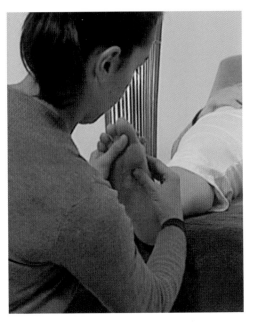

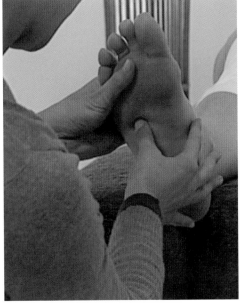

This reflex zone is relaxed by massaging the arch of the foot.

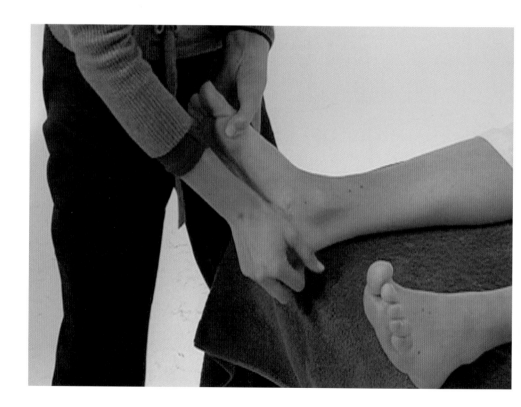

The bile duct reflex zone is also found on the top of the foot. It is always located in the middle of the waist line and the diaphragm line, between zone three and four. Pressure is applied gently using the index finger.

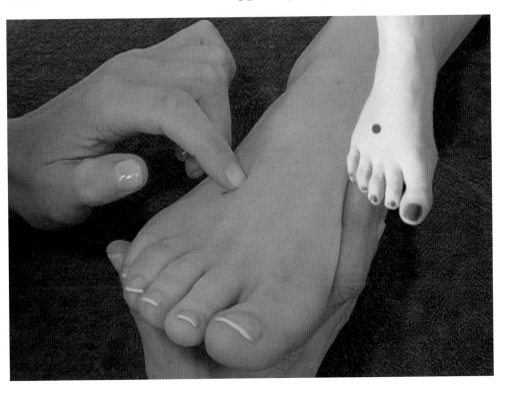

The small intestine reflex zone is situated between the heel line and the waist line.

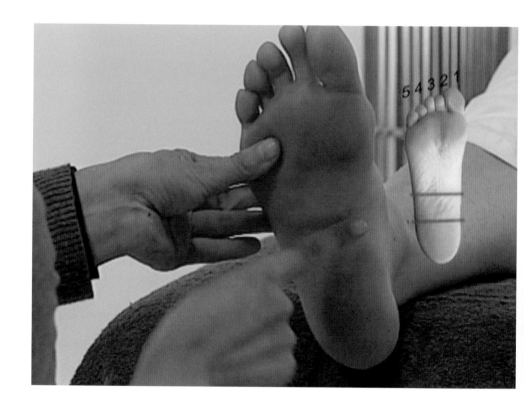

Creeping thumb movements crossing diagonally from the waist line to the diaphragm line are used to treat this area. It is important to start work on the intestine with the right foot, so that the treatment follows the logical way in which foodstuffs travel down the digestive tracts. One or two movements forwards and back can be carried out on this reflex zone.

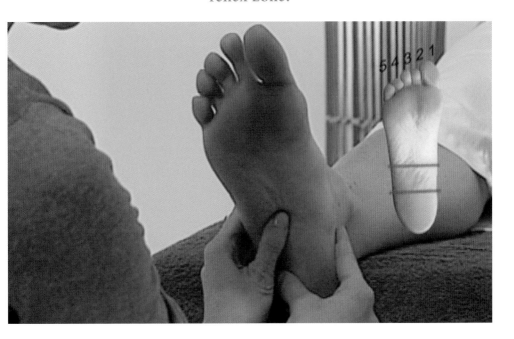

The section of the colon going upwards can be found on the outer edge of the right foot, between the heel line and the waist line and in zone 5.

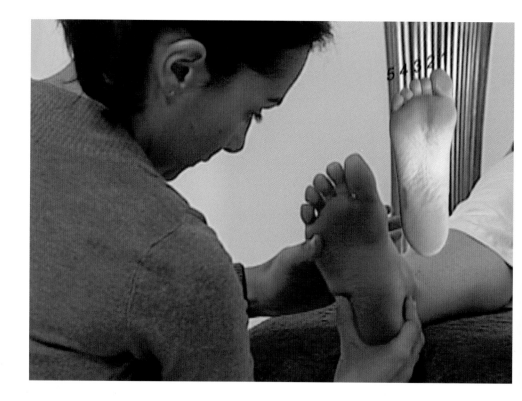

Treatment is administered from the bottom up and one or two movements are sufficient.

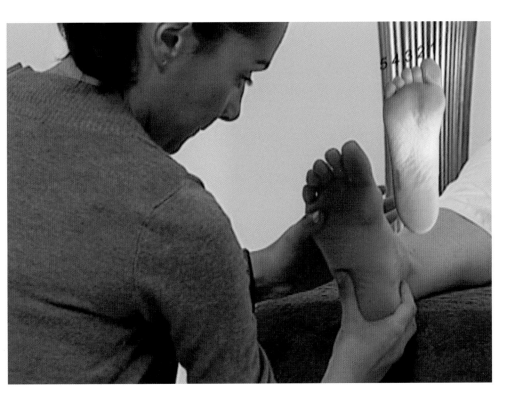

The section of the colon that goes across is found at the lower edge of the waist line on both feet. Creeping thumb movements from the outer edge towards the inner edge are used to treat this area.

Step 1

Step 2

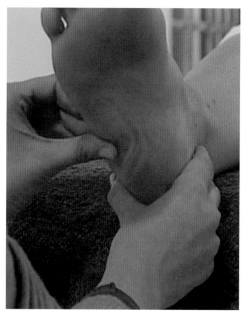

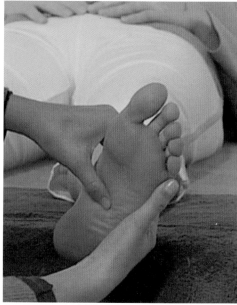

As the colon goes further across it is reflected in the left foot and the treatment is carried out by moving from the inner edge this time to the outer edge, unlike the right foot.

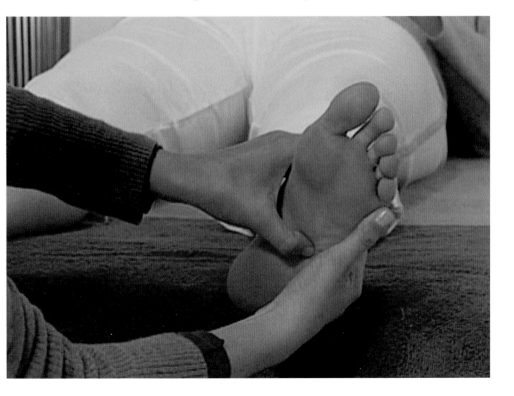

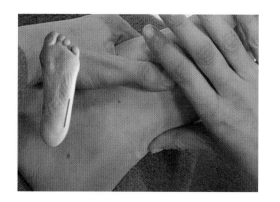

The reflex zone for the colon travelling downwards is found on the outer edge of the left foot at the sigmoid point on the waist line.

When you arrive at the sigmoid point it is beneficial to press down a couple of times.

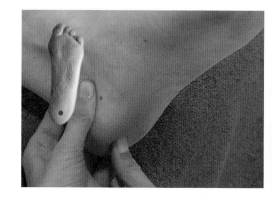

This reflex zone is then followed by work on the rectum. This is found on the line running from the sigmoid point to the point where the heel line reaches the edge of the foot.

Step 1

Step 2

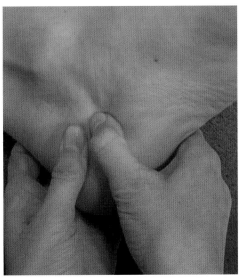
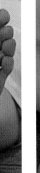

Zones reflecting the digestive system are treated in cases of vomiting, stomach ulcers, colitis, and other problems relating to digestion.

Chapter 7

The Vertebral Column

Neck muscles are reflected in the zone between the base of the toenail and the toe.

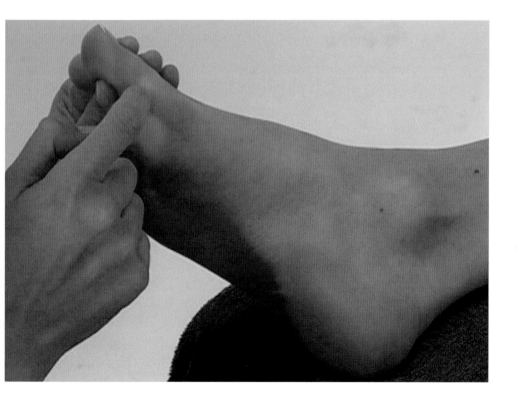

Back muscles between the base of the toe and the waist line.

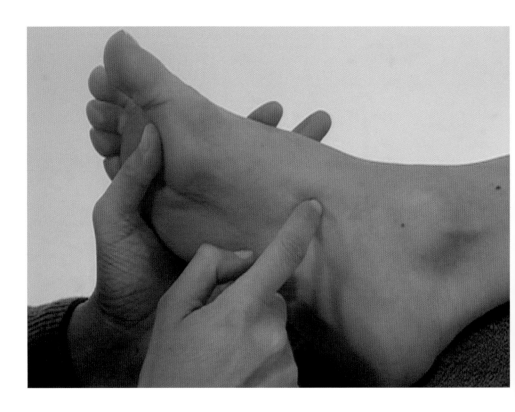

Lumbar muscles between the waist line and the heel line. The reflex zone for the lumbar muscles supplies the nerves for the bladder, the small intestine and the colon.

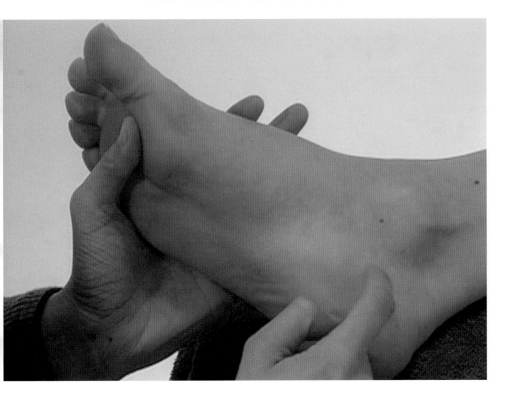

And the zone for the sacrum and the coccyx are between the heel line and the back of the heel.

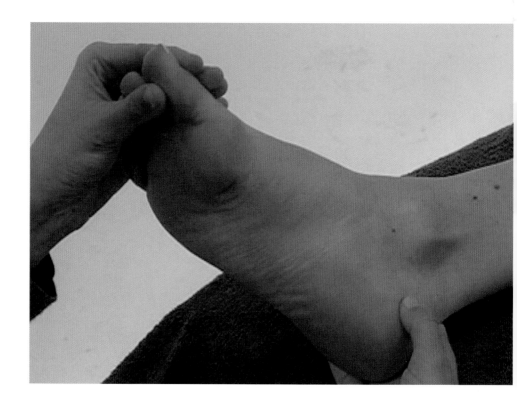

Creeping thumb movements are used to treat the vertebral column reflex zone and the patient's foot is held by the toes using the other hand. One or more forward and backward movements can be carried out on this area. It is treated for cases of neuralgia, the back, neck and lumbar muscles. It is also useful for cases of stress.

Step 1

Step 2

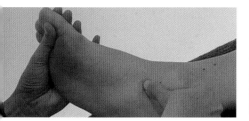
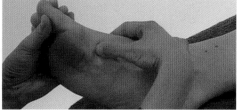

Step 3

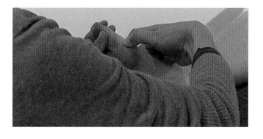

When it comes to the reflex zone relating to the neck muscles, it is best to use the index finger as opposed to the thumb because this zone is more sensitive and much smaller. The neck muscle reflex zone is an important zone because it is also the reflex zone for the optic, olfactory and auditory nerves.

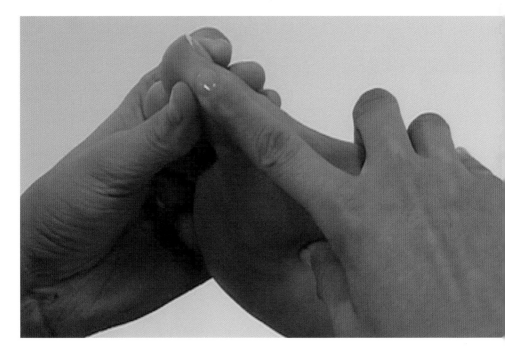

Relaxation of the vertebral column is achieved by twisting movements. The hands are placed side-by-side, parallel with the line running from the metatarsal to the flanges of the first metatarsal and with the palms in contact with the top of the foot and the thumbs level with the foot arch. A twisting movement is carried out on the foot by the hand nearest the big toe. The other hand keeps quite still during the movement. Both hands then need to move towards the toes so that treatment is given across the entire area. At least two or three twisting movements are applied in each zone.

Step 1

Step 2

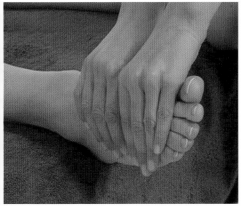
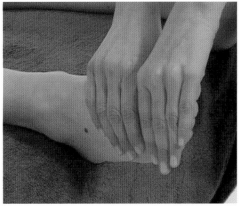

Chapter 8

The Urinary System

The bladder's reflex zone can be found on both feet at the intersection between the heel line and the vertebral column's reflex zone. Creeping thumb movements moving upwards on the diagonal over an area of some 2 square centimetres are used to treat this zone. One can move over and back several times in this zone whenever there is any sign of swelling or congestion, but otherwise it is enough to go over the area once and back.

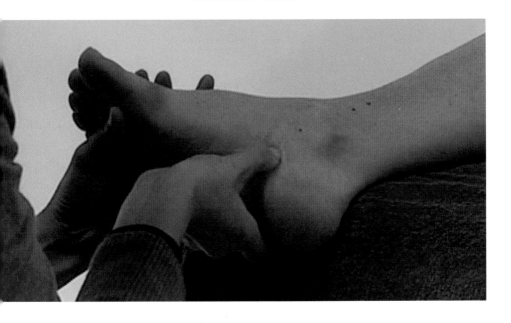

The urethra's reflex zone is situated on the inner edge of the ligament line right up to the waist line.

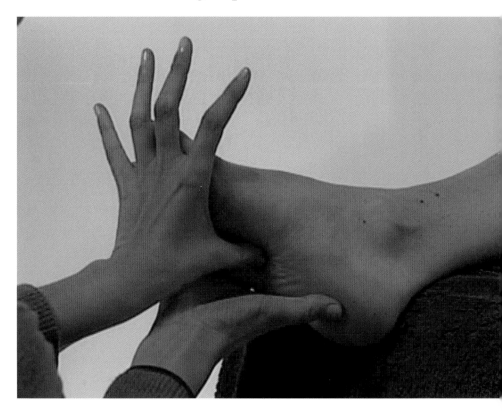

The kidney's reflex zone occurs on both feet, level with the waist line and on the outer edge of the ligament line. It is worked vertically in both directions, but it can also be worked going across.

Step 1

Step 2

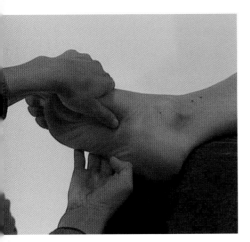
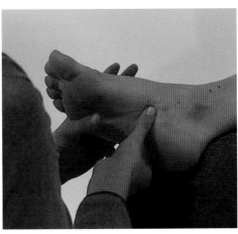

After working on the kidney's reflex zone a return to the urethra is necessary, followed by further work on the bladder zone. The reflex zones relating to the urinary system are worked in cases of cystitis, renal colic, shingles, incontinence and fatigue.

Design and artwork by Scott Giarnese

Published by Demand Media Limited

Publishers Jason Fenwick & Jules Gammond

Written by Michelle Brachet